C000088664

THE ELIMINATION DIET

A 9-WEEK PLAN TO IDENTIFY NEGATIVE FOOD TRIGGERS, GET BETTER GUT HEALTH, GET RID OF BLOATING & BRAIN FOG, AND LIVE A HEALTHIER LIFE.

TODD STRONG   D.C. DACNB, CFMP, PAK

WWW.STRONGHEALTHINSTITUTE.COM

LIMITS OF LIABILITY/DISCLAIMER OF WARRANTY

This book is designed to be a helpful educational resource for the reader. The Author and Publisher, Dr. Todd Strong, makes no representation or warranties with respect to the accuracy, applicability, fitness or completeness of the contents of this program. They accept no liability of any kind for any losses or damages caused or alleged to be caused directly or indirectly, from using the information contained in this book.

This book is not intended for use as a source of any legal or medical advice. Please note that the information contained in this book may be subject to varying international, federal, state and/or local laws or regulations. The purchaser or reader of this publication assumes responsibility for the use of these materials and information.

All information is intended for your general knowledge only and is not a substitute for medical advice or treatment for specific medical conditions. You should seek prompt medical care for any specific health issues and consult your physician before starting a new fitness regimen.

Copyright © 2020 Dr. Todd Strong

All rights reserved worldwide

Dr. Todd Strong owns all rights, titles, and interests in this publication. No part of this book may be reproduced, distributed, or transmitted in any form, in whole or in part, or by any means, mechanical or electronic, including photocopying and recording, or by any information storage and retrieval system, or transmitted by email, without permission in writing from the Publisher.

Disclaimer Notice:

Please note the information contained within this document is for educational and entertainment purposes only. All effort has been executed to present accurate, up to date, and reliable, complete information. No warranties of any kind are declared or implied. Readers acknowledge that the author is not engaging in the rendering of legal, financial, medical or professional advice. The content within this book has been derived from various sources. Please consult a licensed professional before attempting any techniques outlined in this book.

By reading this document, the reader agrees that under no circumstances is the author responsible for any losses, direct or indirect, which are incurred as a result of the use of the information contained within this document, including, but not limited to, — errors, omissions, or inaccuracies.

A FREE GIFT TO OUR READERS!

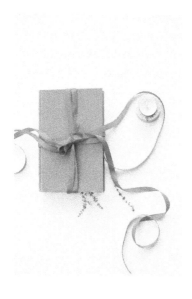

Get our *free* "**Elimination Diet Starter Pack**" with done-for-you templates, **food checklists**, a downloadable **food diary**, and more!

If you want to make your Elimination Diet experience as easy and successful as possible, then you should get these materials right now!

Visit this link:

https://stronghealthinstitute.activehosted.com/f/19

CONTENTS

INTRODUCTION

Hi, this is Dr. Todd Strong. I'm a functional medicine practitioner based out of Cookeville, TN, and I am really excited you found this book.

It can change your life, if you let it.

I wrote this book to demonstrate how effective an elimination diet can be and how anyone from the comfort of their home can experience the benefits of running an elimination diet experiment, as long as they have the will and desire to stick through it.

There isn't any fluff. We don't spend forever on small details or go way too far into the science behind irritants, allergies, and other theories around food. Instead, it's designed to give you exactly what you need to try the elimination diet for yourself. No more, no less.

If you're struggling to find answers to why you can't escape brain fog, chronic pain, fatigue, bloating, gas, diarrhea, headaches, inability to lose weight, or any other frustrating issues that are preventing you from living the life you'd like, then you're going to want to read this book carefully and thoroughly. The elimination diet isn't a miracle cure, but it is the best tool we have to figure out if underlying food sensitivities are the reasons for your symptoms and rebuild your diet into something that serves you and makes you feel good, instead of the other way around.

I'm excited to hear about the life-changing results you experience.

1

HOW TWO MONTHS OF PURPOSEFUL EATING WILL CHANGE YOUR LIFE FOREVER

"My mother told me later that she felt that I might die soon..."

Leanne was at the lowest point of her life. She was depressed, had chronic pain, and was living without hope. She had a desperate desire to feel better. How had she managed to get so unhealthy in just a few short years? She ran several races in her early 30s — even finishing a half marathon! Now, she was sitting in an office at the Strong Health Institute talking about how her quality of life and physical health had fallen apart.

She wasn't sleeping well, she had daily migraines, her face, hands, and feet were so swollen she was

embarrassed to be seen in public... Her blood pressure was way over, she had a complete lack of energy, and she gained 30lbs in a year and a half. In 2017, she had an MRI that showed lesions on her brain and was told it appeared to be Multiple Sclerosis. **She was 38 and didn't expect to live much longer...**Her own kids were taking care of her as she lay bed-ridden. They didn't deserve that responsibility, but they stepped up.

No doctors or medication seemed to help. She was trying everything, and all she wanted was relief. After a careful analysis of her nutritional profile & medical history, Dr. Strong recommended an elimination diet cleanse plan coupled with supplements designed to balance out her nutritional intake. What did she have to lose? She dove in, and she noticed *immediately* how she **felt more refreshed**in the morning, **had more energy**,and **started losing weight**.*Her joints felt better, her hands and feet weren't swollen, her headaches became less frequent, and her blood pressure came down to the normal range.* **She started feeling hope again.**

The second phase of the elimination diet program reintroduces foods and switches up the supplements. As she began this second phase, she began feeling well enough to begin going for walks. **9 months later, she now lives a life**

of restful sleep, no anxiety, no migraines, normal blood pressure, and no chronic pain. Leannehas also lost 50 lbsand is completely off prescription medications. *Her children are so thankful to have their mom back...*

Does any of Leanne's story speak to you? The frantic searching for health? The symptoms — be it chronic fatigue, bloating, weight gain, or lack of energy? If so, then you're in the right place. **Leanne found a way out, and I'm going to show it to you in this book.**

My name is Dr. Todd Strong, and I get what you're going through. I really do. I grew up in a very small town with hard-working parents. I was given everything I could have asked for growing up. All the cookies, candies, TV, and video games a child could dream of. My understanding of health was nonexistent, and my parents grew up in the hills of Tennessee with little to no sugary foods, labored outside everyday, and had no TV. They were both healthy and were giving their child everything they didn't have growing up. By the time I reached the age of 11, I was roughly 200 lbs — only five pounds less than I weigh today.

Believe me, I was not a muscle-packed 11-year-old either. Not that I'm particularly built now, but you know what I mean. Being obese is difficult. You deal with self-conscious feelings, social awkwardness, and depression. It took a serious toll on my psyche, as I'm sure some of you are familiar with. For me, the breakthrough moment was the summer I decided to eliminate sugar and inflammatory foods for two months. In just a few short weeks, I was feeling physically and mentally stronger than I ever had before, and I haven't looked back since.

I'm about to say something you may be sick of, but stick with me and it will all make sense. *If you choose to change your diet, you will change your life.*In the other words, the answers you're searching for are **still**likely in the food you're eating. It's easy to get exhausted with diets. There's Keto, Whole30, Atkins, Paleo, FMD — you name it, and each of these comes with its own theories on what works and what doesn't.

The issue is,**popular diets are fundamentally a generalized approach**,and we're all different, right? Our bodies react differently to different types of food. If they didn't, allergies wouldn't exist! In other words, **a diet plan that works for one person isn't guaranteed to work as well for someone else**,and that's a nutritional fact that is ignored by many diet experts & programs. The solution? You need to identify which foods are working for and against YOU. Then, and *only* then, can you build out a list of foods and diet programs you can rely on to reach your health goals.

That's where the Elimination Diet comes in.

The Elimination Diet is the only diet that takes your unique health responses into account

The Elimination Diet isn't really a traditional "diet" at all — it's a rotating experiment designed to figure out which foods your body reacts well and poorly to and why. Imagine

this scenario: let's say you've been experimenting with a diet that recommends full-fat Greek Yogurt, but you've been feeling bloated and a little sick ever since you started. You assume that this is just the natural side effects of your change in eating habits, but what if it wasn't? What if you were just lactose intolerant? You would never know until you purposely excluded dairy and analyzed how you felt.

That's the Elimination Diet in a nutshell — by isolating food groups, types, and habits, you can build a profile of ideal foods & eating habits for YOU. Not for anyone else. For you. It's the best method bar none for figuring out sensitivities, allergies, and food intolerances. It's the only way to know if food is what's causing your inflammation, fatigue, gas, bloating, and other symptoms.

Think of the power of that. If you knew that dairy made you feel bloated, carbs are fine in moderation but leave you feeling lethargic if you eat them every day, and that red meat kept you up if you ate it past 8 o'clock at night, wouldn't that empower you to make smarter eating choices?

THE HIDDEN BENEFIT OF THE ELIMINATION DIET

No amount of reading diet books or smart food planning can replace analyzing your

own body's reactions to food groups. Think of the Elimination Diet as your "research" and other diets as your "application". Unlike other diets, the elimination diet gives you something special: the unique knowledge of how your body and gut reacts to foods.

Once you complete the elimination diet, you can use that knowledge to make an educated decision on what diet or nutrition plan is best suited for your goals *and* your body. Think of it like the foundation you need *before* you try other diets. If you've been struggling with eating well and sticking to diets, then this is the piece you've been missing.

The Elimination Diet isn't hard — if you have a plan.

Don't worry if the elimination diet sounds intimidating. That's exactly what this book will solve. I'm going to show you exactly how to conduct a safe elimination diet test and give you the actionable steps you can take to start your elimination diet journey today.It's not long, but every bit of it is important. If you take the time to read this book completely, you'll have the best chance to determine what foods may be the root cause of your issues & discover how to live free from the distress you're experiencing.

This book gives you everything you need, but if you prefer professional guidance and accountability, don't hesitate to reach out. We help people finally solve their chronic symptoms every day, and nothing makes me happier than seeing those lightbulb moments. You can contact me here: https://stronghealthinstitute.com/

I also encourage you to grab our Elimination Diet starter pack that we use in-house, free of charge, which you can use to track your progress and analyze your results. It makes the whole process easy to understand and execute. More on that later, though.

Let's go!

2

WHY "COMMON" FOODS CAN'T ALWAYS BE TRUSTED

"(My experience) was weeks of clean eating and understanding what I was putting in my body. It was hard at first but it was giving me a chance to improve my quality of life with food and not medicine. I noticed a difference shortly after starting and haven't fallen or had trouble walking ever since. I tell everyone about what helped me and wouldn't be where I am with my health without the knowledge and insight of Dr. Todd Strong."

It can be easy to sound like a conspiracy theorist when discussing nutrition, but believe me — you can respect science and distrust public opinion at the same time, and there's no clearer example than the "fats are bad" nutrition campaigns that ran for over half of the 20th century. They were a disastrous bungling of our public health, and we're still dealing with the fallout.

Take a look at this excerpt from April 2008's Oxford Academic:

"By the 1960s, the low-fat diet began to be touted not just for high-risk heart patients, but as good for the whole nation. After 1980, the low-fat approach became an overarching ideology, promoted by physicians, the federal government, the food industry, and the popular health media.

Many Americans subscribed to the ideology of low fat, even though there was no clear evidence that it prevented heart disease or promoted weight loss.

Ironically, in the same decades that the low-fat approach assumed ideological status, Americans in the aggregate were getting fatter, leading to what many called an obesity epidemic.

Nevertheless, the low-fat ideology had such a hold on Americans that skeptics were dismissed. Only recently has evidence of a paradigm shift begun to surface, first with the challenge of the low-carbohydrate diet and then, with a more moderate approach, reflecting recent scientific knowledge about fats."

Throughout that period, soda lobbyists were fully onboard with the low-fat ideology. Why? Because it took focus away from **sugar**,which most of us now know is much more widespread and damaging than fats could ever be. To elaborate a bit, studies have shown that sugar is actually the cause of heart disease and not cholesterol. Sugar inflames your blood vessels, and then your body reacts to that inflammation by producing cholesterol to patch and heal those inflamed blood vessels. That cholesterol begins to build on the artery walls, which gradually decreases the room your blood has to flow and eventually culminates into fatal heart attacks and other diseases.

As you can see from this example, correlation does not always mean causation. Sugar is the root cause and cholesterol gets the blame for doing it's job. So what's the point?

*We're seeing a similar slowness and public awareness transition with food allergies and intolerances,*and there is widespread evidencethat common foods we take for granted are having significant effects on our health, sense of wellbeing, and longevity.

Allow me to explain...

FOOD INTOLERANCES ARE RAMPANT

While around 4%of American adults have allergies, an estimated 15-20%of adults have food intolerances and sensitivities. That figure covers everything from lactose intolerances, to reactions to additives like food colorings or sulfites, to malabsorption of nutrients. With up to 1 in 5 people having an intolerance, isn't it likely that you could be eating multiple foods that are stirring up these intolerances and contributing to your health issues?

Food intolerances are rising

The problem isn't getting better, either. Recent epidemiological surveys demonstrate that a rapid increase in allergic diseases is a legitimate issue. In developing countries, examples of widespread allergies and intolerances can affect up to 30%of the population.

So what can we do to identify these intolerances and make smarter food choices that have the potential to eliminate damaging chronic symptoms like fatigue and bloating? We can use the best tool we have: The Elimination Diet.

Through straightforward elimination and experimentation, we can find out the common foods that may be causing your health issues. And that doesn't mean eating will be boring after your elimination diet, it just means that you'll have the information you need to indulge when you want and feel healthy when you want.

In the next chapter, we'll be looking a bit more at why the Elimination Diet works so well and who it works best for. After that, we'll dive into the specifics.

3

WHAT THE ELIMINATION DIET CAN DO FOR YOU & WHO SHOULD TRY IT

The secret weapon for fighting back against food intolerances & allergies

Note: The elimination diet is an altering of your nutritional habits, so if you have underlying conditions or suspect you are highly allergic to certain foods, please do not conduct an elimination diet without a professional physician.

WHAT MAKES THE ELIMINATION DIET SUCH A POWERFUL TOOL?

Elimination diets are the "gold standard" for identifying food intolerances, sensitivities, and allergies through diet.

You may be asking, "why?" Aren't allergy tests already doing that? In part, yes, but there is a flaw: Many people have years of chronic exposure to foods they are sensitive to. This causes the body to adapt to a low level state of inflammation that is slowly causing physiological changes, including arthritis, autoimmune, fatigue, etc. And due to the ability of the body to adapt, food allergies tests do not take into account immune adaptations but rather only test a baseline of "normal" ranges from your particular demographic.

In other words, our body's ability to adapt can blind traditional allergy tests.

This is why the gold standard for diagnosis remains the double-blind, placebo-controlled food challenge. The benefits of the elimination diet have been proven for a variety of diseases as well:

The science showing the benefits of elimination-style diets for treating IBS, dermatitis, adult eosinophilic esophagitis (EoE), and ADHD is extremely strong.

For example, a 2005 study in the Journal of the American College of Nutrition demonstratedthat using the elimination diet for IBS patients who didn't respond to standard therapy results saw significant impacts on overall wellbeing and quality of life, and a separate 2014 study by the Journal of Clinical and Aesthetic Dermatology linked

elimination diets to a decrease in dermatitis. There is also a list of resources and studies at the end of this eBook if you'd like to do more research.

THE LIFE-CHANGING BENEFITS OF THE ELIMINATION DIET

Now, let's get specific by covering the benefits and risks of an elimination diet & who should and shouldn't try it.

The primary benefits of an Elimination Diet

It gives you the priceless knowledge of what foods affect you negatively

If you struggle from chronic and fleeting bouts of symptoms, then this could be the way out for you. By understanding what foods affect you and how, you have the power to choose how the food you eat makes you feel. This switch is life-changing and cannot be stressed enough.

May reduce IBS symptoms

Because many of the foods eliminated during the clean phase are known to be irritants, such as sugar, processed carbohydrates, and preservatives, the elimination diet by default reduces intestinal irritation and gives your body the time and positive probiotics it needs to begin repairing itself.

May reduce ADHD

Studiesfound in the National Library of Medicine have shown that in "young children with ADHD an elimination diet can lead to a statistically significant decrease in symptoms." If you have a child who isn't responding well to medication, then trying an elimination diet may be worth it.

It May Help People With Eosinophilic Esophagitis

Eosinophilic Esophagitis, or EoE, is an inflammatory disease that affects the esophagus, or the tube that connects your mouth to your stomach. When people with EoE eat foods they are allergic or sensitive to, it can worsen EoE and further restrict their esophagus, making it difficult to swallow among other symptoms.

Because the elimination diet removes top allergenic foods in their entirety, studies have shown that this diet can help manage EoE and improve the lives of people who take this diet to heart. For example, a study by the Journal of Allergy and Clinical Immunology found that forty-nine (73.1%) patients exhibited significantly reduced eosinophil peak counts before reintroducing those foods back into their diet, and more importantly, **found that all patients who**

continued to avoid the offending foods maintained histopathologic and clinical EoE remission for up to 3 years. That's amazing.

It May Improve Skin Conditions Like Eczema

Again, research by Journal of Clinical and Aesthetic Dermatology has found that dietary factors can exacerbate dermatitis, which causes skin rashes and itching.

May help with migraines

Using the elimination diet to identify common migraine triggers like chocolate, alcohol, and dairy products is well documented.

WHO IS THE ELIMINATION DIET FOR?

While the elimination diet is not for everyone, there are many people who can benefit from this experiment. If you've been on and off medication, suffer chronic pain, have doctor after doctor telling you to just exercise and eat healthy but nothing seems to work, then you may be exactly who this diet is best for.

More specifically, if you're suffering from:

- Chronic fatigue

- Weight gain
- Digestive issues
- Headaches
- Gas/bloating
- Mental fog
- Hormonal issues
- Aching joints or arthritis.
- Diarrhea or other issues with your stools.

And aren't sure where to turn and haven't conducted an elimination diet in the past, then you're in the right place.

WHO IS THE ELIMINATION DIET NOT FOR?

Let me be very clear here: the Elimination Diet is *not*for everyone.

Think of it as a tool that we can use to test whether or not certain foods may be decreasing the quality of our lives. Many people have food allergies and sensitivities that they may not be aware of, and they are great candidates for the elimination diet — but it is not a catch-all diet and isn't the most appropriate choice for people in many situations.

So who shouldn't go on the Elimination Diet? Here are a few categories:

- Pregnant women
- People suffering from acute illnesses or diseases
- People only looking to lose weight (the Elimination Diet is **not** a traditional diet!)
- Individuals with a history of malnutrition or eating disorders.

And another important note: If you have or suspect you have an anaphylactic or recognized food allergy, ***do not conduct reintroduction without a trained healthcare professional.*** If you've been avoiding a certain food because you suspect a strong allergy and then reintroduce it as a test, this can put your health at risk. And more generally, if you're unsure if you qualify, then you should consult with a health professional.

The risks of an Elimination Diet

Like any substantial lifestyle change, there are risks if you don't approach the elimination diet with the care it deserves. This is why it's so helpful to hire a professional to guide you through, but here are a few things to be wary of:

It can put you at risk of nutritional deficiencies if you don't use supplements or pay careful attention to your nutrition.

The clean phase is fairly drastic. You are cutting out almost all sugars, carbs, preservatives, many grains, dairy products, etc. It's possible you've been using some of these categories to supply certain vitamins and minerals, and by eliminating them from your diet you could run low on some of the nutrients you need.

One way to avoid this issue is supplements. I use supplements and vitamins to make sure my clients are still getting a balanced nutritional intake during their clean phase, and I'd be happy to point you in the right direction when you're ready to begin your elimination diet.

Children and adults may experience social anxiety as a result of the diet.

Because the diet is substantial, you or your child may experience social pressure and anxiety as a result of their new eating habits. This is difficult to avoid but should be recognized so you can provide support.

Why are there so many types of Elimination Diets?

If you've been doing a bit of searching around the elimination diet world, you may have noticed that there are many types of elimination diets. There's the low-FODMAP elimination diet, the rare foods elimination diet, the few foods elimination diet, the fasting elimination diet, among others. In fact, even diets like gluten-free, sugar-free, and lactose-free diets are technically a simple form of an elimination diet. Remember that the elimination diet is a tool we have to test how our bodies react to certain foods. It isn't for everyone, and some versions of the elimination diet are better for some people over others — but this is typically because they are already aware of certain sensitivities or have specific medical conditions.

WHAT KIND OF ELIMINATION DIET IS COVERED IN THIS BOOK?

The elimination diet I cover in this eBook is a generalized approach. It's for people who don't have a lot of information to work from and are tired of running in circles and not knowing what diet or treatment is best for them. It's a "clean slate" approach to figuring out what foods are affecting you and why. With this in mind, you may notice that my version of the elimination diet allows some foods that others don't and vice versa. This is nothing to worry about. If you take the time to complete the elimination diet in this book, your health will thank you. In the next chapter, we're going to start covering some specifics on what the Elimination Diet looks like and a few tips for making it a success.

4

OVERVIEW & TIPS FOR RUNNING A SUCCESSFUL ELIMINATION DIET

"The doctor of the future will give no medicine, but will interest his patient in the care of the human frame, in diet and in the cause and prevention of disease."

— THOMAS EDISON

THE ELIMINATION DIET: THE PLAN & HOW IT WORKS

The elimination diet is *fundamentally* short-term.

Think of it as a short sprint. Once you finish, you'll have concrete information on what foods make *you* feel what way and why. *You.* No one else. And you know what else is great? That "uniquely yours" information will serve you for the rest of your life. If you do the work now, you'll reap the benefits for decades to come. My patients' lives are being changed every day by this approach, and I'm so excited to hear your story and transformation — you're going to do great — and more importantly, *feel* great!

The entire process varies in length but typically takes around 7-10 weeks to get all of the information you need.

It's split up like this, and we cover all of these phases in detail in the following chapter.

ELIMINATION DIET GENERAL STRUCTURE

Phase #1: Preparation

Duration: 1-2 Days

This is when you take a few days to review the steps you need to take, organize your food diary, plan your weeks, etc.

Phase #2: Establishing your health foundation

Duration: 1 week

This is when you track your normal eating habits and symptoms over a week, making note of what you feel and when. This will serve as your foundation to compare back to after your experiment is over.

Phase #3: Cleaning Phase

Duration: 3 weeks

3 weeks of clean eating, where we safely eliminate as many potential irritants as possible.*The stricter you eat, the better your results will be.*

In other words, the best elimination diets are the most restricting. This is the hardest but most rewarding part of the elimination diet. You'll be surprised by what you learn to love and hate during this period.

Phase #4: Gradual Reintroduction & Evaluation

Duration: 5-6 weeks

This is when you slowly introduce potential irritants food by food, taking 5 days to carefully analyze how you feel upon reintroduction. This is when we really start discovering what food makes you feel what ways and why. This is my favorite part of the process, and I can't wait for you to experience it for yourself.

Phase #5: A return to your "new" normal

Duration: A lifetime!

At this point in the process, you'll know how various foods affect you, and you can build your lifestyle around those triggers. You are going to feel so empowered with the knowledge you gain from this experience. That's it! That's all that stands between you and a life where *you* get to choose how you feel instead of food choosing for you. If you start to get overwhelmed, don't worry! Plenty of people are changing their lives with the elimination diet, and you can too! By using the diet lists and best practices, a lot of the thinking is done for you. All you have to do is commit. With that in mind, here's a summary list of what you CAN'T eat during the "clean phase".

We also have a more specific and printable version that you can download in our free starter pack.

Get that by going here:

https://stronghealthinstitute.activehosted.com/f/19

WHAT YOU CAN'T EAT DURING THE 3-WEEK "CLEAN PHASE".

Instead of trying to memorize this whole list, it helps to think of the big picture. In general, the closer you can get to all-natural vegetables and lean meats, the better. If you fill up most of your grocery cart with fresh vegetables and fruits, then you're on the right track. Then, think of the obvious culprits you know you shouldn't be eating anyway. That means sugar, carbs, dairy, alcohol, frozen foods, etc. Your vices have to go, and we're trying to get as far away from preservatives as possible.

More specifically, you can't have:

- Any dairy milk and alternative milk products, excluding coconut and rice milks.
- Protein powders.
- Large amounts of sugary fruits like strawberries.
- Soups (unless they're homemade!)
- Alcohol.
- Nuts and Seeds (refer to diagram on page 56)
- Corn.
- All breads (with the exclusion of small portions of fresh sourdough)
- Ketchups, sauces, and other preservative-filled spreads.

- Salad dressings.
- Milk and white chocolates.
- Frozen foods (always filled with preservatives and irritants)

See? It's most of what you would expect. These are the most common culprits that people are allergic to, so avoiding the extra muck that companies put in food to preserve shelf life is most of the list. Unfortunately, irritants and problem ingredients can be found in lots of unexpected places, so here are a few ingredients to know of as you scan those food labels.

Typical culprits & irritants to watch out for

While everyone's body reacts to certain foods differently, we do know the most common culprits that negatively affect health. These are most commonly *carbohydrates* and their most common form — sugars.

Additives & ingredients to watch out for on food labels:

- **Lactose**(a.k.a. Milk sugar). You find lactose in dairy products like milk, yogurt, cream, etc.
- **Fructose**(a.k.a. Fruit sugar). You can find this in snack foods and drinks the world over, but it also includes honey, molasses, agave, syrups, etc.

- **Carrageenan.**This is an irritant food additive made from seaweed.
- **Soy & MSG**(monosodium glutamate). This is most often found in Asian foods and sauces, cheap snacks, and other processed foods. Eating fresh should exclude your risk here, but it's always good to keep an eye out!
- **Wheat**(excluding homemade sourdough bread).
- **Chicory root, inulin, fructo-oligosaccharides.**
- **Sorbitol, xylitol, or hydrogenated starch hydrolysates.**

WHAT YOU CAN EAT DURING THE 3-WEEK "CLEAN PHASE".

Now, let's talk about what you can eat. It's absolutely possible to eat well during the elimination diet. Some of you are shaking your head, but believe me! How does slow-roasted salmon with asparagus and roasted squash sound? Or shredded chicken with cashew rice? See? It's not all bad.

Here's what you CAN eat during the 3-week "Clean Phase".

- All fruits except citrus fruits like limes and lemons.
- All vegetables.

- Alternative milks like coconut milk and rice milk.
- Teas and water.
- Lean meats like chicken and turkey.
- Lamb
- Salmon
- Olive oil, coconut oil, and flaxseed oil.
- Spices excluding cayenne pepper and paprika.
- Distilled vinegar.
- Rice
- Buckwheat

WHAT THINGS YOU NEED TO HAVE TO SUCCEED WITH AN ELIMINATION DIET

You don't need much at all to make a life-changing impact. There isn't any special equipment required other than what you already have around the house. That's part of what makes this experiment so great for people all around the world.

All you need is:

- Access to fresh vegetables, meat, and water.
- A notebook, computer, or phone to use as a food diary.
- The desire to get healthy!

That's it! Anything else you spend money on are just ways to have accountability and make it easier on yourself. For example, if you'd rather play it safe, have accountability, and let someone guide you through the process to ensure you finish it, then <u>working with</u> a health professionalis the best choice! That costs money, sure, but it's often worth it to make sure you actually finish what you started. Now, let's get into the details.

5

THE STEP-BY-STEP, 5-PHASE GUIDE TO RUNNING AN ELIMINATION DIET

This chapter is the exact process you need to take to finish an elimination diet and track your results. If you follow this advice to the letter, you will succeed.

Okay. Let's begin.

PHASE #1: PREPARATION

Duration: 1 Day

Goal: To make the next few weeks as easy as possible

Phase 1 is all about making the next few weeks easier on yourself.

Take the time to prepare your grocery list, recipes, and expectations. Using this time to prepare is what separates people who manage to get through an elimination diet and those who don't. It's natural to feel a little funny or weak when adjusting your diet, so you want to remove as many hurdles as possible before you hit the go button.

Here's exactly how to start:

Step #1 - Get in the right headspace

Take a moment to recognize that changing your diet isn't easy, but you know it will be worth it. Accept that there will be moments you won't like or enjoy. Take stock in knowing that the elimination diet is not forever, but the impact it can have your life can be. An example would be when you are about to go on a hard hike or take a run — you know the journey will be tough but the rewards will make it all worth it.

Step #2 - Ask your friends and family for accountability

While the elimination diet is a personal endeavor, it's much easier to finish when your friends and family are supporting you. Let them know what you're up to and how long

you'll be on the diet. The fewer times you feel pressured to eat certain foods or go out with friends, the easier it will be to succeed. Remind them also that this is temporary, and if the diet is successful they may get to spend even more quality time with you in the future. If you aren't dealing with chronic symptoms, then you will be able to spend more time doing what you love with your family. Help them help you!

Step #3 - Decide if you're going to work with a professional

Having a health professional to guide you through the elimination diet is a fantastic use of your time and money. If you want to ensure that your elimination diet journey is a success, then this is the surefire route. It's like hiring a personal trainer. Sure, you don't *need* one to work out, but are they amazing for accountability, education, and direction? Of course. And functional medicine practitioners are the best choice for something like the Elimination Diet because we focus on the root issues. Instead of "Not Sick" care, we understand the complex metabolic processes that help you resolve your issues for good instead of just covering them up with medication.

Step #4 - Get your kitchen Elimination Diet Ready

Part of staying motivated is knowing what you can and can't eat and having a stocked kitchen.**Look over the eat and can't eat lists, check out some elimination diet recipes, and stock your kitchen with *simple* foods and snacks.** The last thing you want to be thinking about when your body is reacting to your change in nutrition is what you can and can't eat.

If you live alone, I recommend moving all of your usual temptations — be it bread, candy, ice cream, whatever out of sight. Don't throw them away if they won't expire over the next few months since we'll be using them during the reintroduction phase, but anything you can do to remove those triggers is ideal. **If you live in a house with other people, then try and designate an area just for you.**That way you can open up the pantry or fridge, look at the second shelf, and know that anything you see is okay to eat.

And remember, while you will be watching the quantities of certain foods you're eating like fruits, the elimination diet is *not* a traditional diet — **meaning you don't have to focus on calorie counting or reducing your serving sizes.**You can get full as long as it's with the right foods. It helps to keep your protein, fat, and fiber content high and avoid eating less than you're used to. By eating less you may drop your blood sugar levels, which

could cause you to confuse your cravings and symptoms of a calorie deficit with negative food associations.

Step #5 - Get your food diary and resources ready

Download the diary sheet here:

https://stronghealthinstitute.
activehosted.com/f/19

Have fun with your food diary & build it into your existing habits

Go ahead and take this time to get your food diary ready. Make *10 weeks* of diaries just to be safe. Not everyone needs this many, but it's best to prepare for it anyway. If you're into journaling, then buying a new notebook or dedicating a section to your food diary is ideal. If you hate writing things down and prefer to use your phone, do that! The point is to make it easy on yourself by tying these new habits to the ones you already have.

There are also a lot of great apps and other digital resources available if you prefer. My app recommendations are:

mySymptoms Food Diary- $3.99

Cara- Free

Deliciously Ella- Free with in-app purchases

You can also load all of the weeks into your Google Calendar. This is a nice way to remember how far along you are and what days you should be introducing foods, etc. For example, if you started on January 1st, you could have:

January 1st - January 7th: Foundation Week (eat like normal)

8th - 14th: Clean Eating Week 1

15th - 21st: Clean Eating Week 2

22nd - 28th: Clean Eating Week 3

29th - Feb. 2nd: Introduce Food #1 (Starches)

Feb. 3rd - Feb. 7th: Introduce Food #2 (Dairy

Feb. 8rd - Feb. 12th: Introduce Food #3 (Legumes)

Etc.! The trick? Build it into whatever system or format you're most likely to use already.

PHASE #2: ESTABLISH YOUR "FOUNDATION"

Duration: One week.

Goal: To take careful note of your normal dietary habits and symptoms

This phase is all about thinking critically about how you feel *now*based on your current eating habits. You already know your general symptoms, but we want to identify when they happen and keep a general log of what you eat so we can compare it to our testing later. Don't change anything yet —

just go through your normal day but start writing down in your **food diary**how you feel and what you ate. This is good practice for what you'll be doing over the next few weeks when you start reintroducing foods. For example, here's a "foundation" style food diary entry:

March 2nd, 2020.

Morning Meals 6AM - 11AM:

John made bacon and eggs, so I ate three eggs, two slices of bacon, and I had my usual toast with margarine and white toast. This was around 9. I felt fine at first but around 10:30 I got bad cramps and had to use the restroom repeatedly.

Afternoon Meals 11AM - 3PM:

I made a simple chicken caesar salad around 12:30 PM. I got a little sleepy like I usually do after lunch but felt okay.

Dinner Meals: 3PM - 10PM

Had pizza for dinner around 7. Felt really bloated and sleepy about an hour afterward. I didn't sleep very well last night, so maybe it's that, but it was delicious!

PHASE #3: EAT "CLEAN" & RECORD HOW YOU FEEL

Duration: 3 Weeks

Goal: To eliminate all possible irritants and other dietary culprits and observe how it makes you feel.

FOOD GROUP	FOOD ALLOWED	FOOD EXCLUDED
Meat , fish, poultry	Chicken, turkey, lamb, cold water fish, duck, wild game	Red meat, processed meats, eggs and egg substitutes
Dairy	Rice, nut milks such as almond and coconut	Milk, cheese, ice cream, yogurt, non-dairy creamers, butter
Legumes	All legumes (beans, lentils)	Soy
Vegetables	All	Creamed or processed
Fruits	Fresh, frozen, juiced	Strawberries and citrus
Starches	Potatoes, rice, buckwheat, millet, quinoa	Gluten and corn containing products (pasta, bread, chips)
Breads/cereals	Any made from rice, quinoa, amaranth, buckwheat, teff, millet, potato	All made from wheat, spelt, kamut, rye, barley, triticale
Soups	Clear, vegetable based	Canned or creamed
Beverages	Fresh or unsweetened fruit/vegetable juices, herbal teas, filtered/spring water	Dairy, coffee/tea, alcohol, citrus, sodas
Fats/oils	Cold/expeller pressed, flax, olive, walnut, sesame	Margarine, shortening, butter and spreads
Nuts/seeds	Almonds, cashews, pecans, flax, pumpkin, sesame, sunflower seeds, and butters from allowed nuts	Peanut, pistachios, peanut butter
Sweeteners	Brown rice syrup, fruit sweeteners, agave nectar, Stevia	Refined brown/white sugar, maple syrup, honey, fructose, molasses, corn syrup

The "clean" phase lasts for around three weeks, and this is where we take a sweeping approach to what nutritionists have identified as the most "problematic" foods. By reducing foods that are known to cause allergies and inflammation &

foods that are suspected of doing the same, we can temporarily eat an extremely low inflammation diet. This is the hardest part, but you can do it.

Unsurprisingly, a lot of these "clean" recommendations will be recognizable. The clear majority of allergic reactions in the United States are caused by peanuts, tree nuts, cow's milk, eggs, soy, wheat, seafood, and shellfish. By eliminating those, we've already eliminated many of the most common culprits. After that, it's getting rid of other foods suspected or proven to be harmful, such as high fructose corn syrup, preservatives, various sugars, soy, non-dairy substitutes, etc.

Again, think lean, think fresh, and think natural.

If your cart is mostly filled with leafy greens like spinach, kale, lettuce, etc., doesn't have red meat or sugary foods, and is free from packaged or frozen foods, you're most of the way there.

I recommend getting foods and meals that are easy to make. You're going to be balancing a lot, so you may not want to cook new things while running the diet, although some of you may look at that as a challenge. For example, before the first week I'd consider poaching and shredding a whole chicken the day before you begin. This will give you a lot of "ready-to-go" lean meat you can eat over greens like arugula, flash grill on a cast iron, or even microwave. Add some green beans and rice, and you have a few meals covered. Stock up on rice and potatoes, too. When you remove red meat or other typical protein sources from your diet, your body tends to get hungry. It's helpful to have a variety of filling food sources nearby, and rice and potatoes are easy and fast ways to have lots of food around the house.

If salads are more your thing, consider making a quinoa salad for the week! Quinoa, salt, pepper, red peppers, onions, olive oil, red wine vinegar, garlic, parsley, and chick-peas — a big batch can last you a week! For snacking, I recommend picking up some almonds, almond butter, celery, apples, bananas, and healthy smoothie options. Anything from the allowed food list is fair game for snacking, but I've found these options to particularly "grab-and-go".

PHASE #4: EVALUATION & REINTRODUCTION PHASE

Duration: 5-6 weeks (one suspected irritant every 5 days)

Goal: Reintroduce suspect foods one-by-one, examine how you feel, and figure out what the best diet is for your unique body.

Phase 4 is the most important phase of all.

This is when you begin testing and noticing what foods make you feel tired, foggy, bloated, etc. The key is to **only** add one group in at a time. If you add in multiple foods, how will you know which ones make you feel bad?

Here are a few short best practices when reintroducing foods into your diet:

- **Start small**.Everyone feels bad if they eat a 2lb tub of fried chicken. Eat moderate portions of the foods you're reintroducing to avoid triggering any severe negative reactions and to make sure you aren't just feeling poorly from overeating.

- **Eat "pure" versions of that food group**.In other words, for dairy, don't eat butterscotch chocolate ice cream with a waffle cone, choose instead to have a bowl of greek yogurt or plain vanilla ice cream. This way you know exactly what you added.

- **If anything weird happens during your reintroduction phase, start over**.If you get sick during a reintroduction phase, then return to the clean eating phase until the sickness passes (assuming there are no nutritional balance considerations). Then, reintroduce that same food again so you can get an idea of what it does.

- **Take it slow, and refer back to your clean eating symptom diary**whenever you feel something. Do you feel just as good when you were eating clean? Okay, great! Then that food is just fine. Do you feel worse? Then make note of it.
- **If you don't feel anything and still feel good after eating the reintroduced food group for five days, then give it the green light!** You can now eat this food and not have anything to worry about.

Once you're ready to begin, I suggest starting at the top of the above list and going down in order. This way you don't get confused and can always figure out how far along you are. So the first five days you would start with adding in some red meat and eggs, the next five you'd add in some dairy, the following five you'll add in soy, etc. Here's that list in order:

Reintroduction #1: Red Meat/Eggs - Red meat, processed meats, eggs, and egg substitutes.

Reintroduction #2: Dairy - Milk, cheese, ice cream, yogurt, non-dairy creamers, butter.

Reintroduction #3: Legumes: - Soy

Reintroduction #4: Vegetables - Creamed or processed vegetables.

Reintroduction #5: Fruits - Strawberries, limes, lemons, and other citrus fruits.

Reintroduction #6: Starches - Pasta, bread, chips, and other gluten and corn-based products.

Reintroduction #7: Breads/cereals - Any bread or cereal made from wheat, spelt, kamut, rye, barley, or triticale.

Reintroduction #8: Soups - Canned or creamed

Reintroduction #9: Beverages - Dairy, coffee/tea, alcohol, citrus, sodas

Reintroduction #10: Fats/oils - Margarine, shortening, butter, and spreads.

Reintroduction #11: Nuts/Seeds - Peanut, pistachios, peanut butter.

Reintroduction #12: Sweeteners - Refined brown/white sugar, maple syrup, honey, fructose, molasses, corn syrup.

If you knock them out one by one and keep close observations throughout your food diary, you will walk away with the tools you need to feel great from food for the rest of your life.

The whole process takes around two months, but it is a journey worth taking, believe me.

And remember that with each reintroduction the process gets easier and more exciting.

PHASE #5: A RETURN TO YOUR (NEW) NORMAL

Duration: The rest of your life!

Goal: To settle into new eating habits that keep you feeling great

Phase #5 is the beginning of your new life. What I like to do at this point with my clients is create a master food list that is unique to the client so they can print out exactly what they learned during their elimination diet. This is perfect to put in two places: your fridge and your phone.

Every time you're curious if eating that piece of carrot cake will make you feel bad or if eating pasta will make you have gas, you can look at your personal one-sheet to remind you. And remember, sometimes the consequence is worth it! A great thanksgiving meal or occasional treat is part of life, and I don't want you to think you have to get rid of those after the elimination diet. It's more about knowing what you're trading when you choose to eat them. Anytime you're shopping and you want to have a week free from symptoms, you can choose from your own personal master food list and create recipes/shop from there.

I encourage you to add to this list overtime. Hopefully by the end of this process your entire approach to food will be different. Every food will make you think about how it makes you feel and whether or not you enjoy that feeling. The more you listen to your body, the better you'll get at consistently eating a diet that is both nutritionally balanced and keeps you feeling good.

6

TYPICAL OUTCOMES OF AN ELIMINATION DIET

I love seeing my patients' feel great again, and the outcomes of a successful elimination diet are always positive. Even if you discover that food isn't the root cause of your symptoms, you can be empowered by that knowledge, and the clean-eating phase typically changes our diets and makes us healthier anyway! It's a win-win scenario. Here are a few outcomes we see in our patients:

You will FEEL better!

That's the whole point, right!? Imagine waking up in the morning and *not* feeling tired or having gas. How great would it be to just *feel normal.*That is what all of this is about. You have enough on your plate, and you don't need your body to stress you out as well. If your body is negatively reacting to foods, you *will* feel better after this experiment.

The knowledge of what foods make YOU feel what way and why.

Imagine this scenario with me: you're at a friend's house for dinner, and they pull out some delicious Ben & Jerry's ice cream. Two weeks earlier, you had finished your elimination diet and have been feeling so much better. Now, during your reintroduction phase you discovered that if you had more than a cup of full-fat ice cream you got terrible gas, but if you just ate a little bit you didn't have any issues. So you ask your friend for just a small portion and you continue enjoying the evening instead of having to leave early due to discomfort. That is the power of a successful elimination diet, and it's within your reach.

The relative strength of the foods that make you feel certain ways

To expand on that point, it's not always just the food that may be causing your issues but the **amount** of that food. You may be able to have maple syrup 1-2 times a week with greek yogurt, but you may not be able to eat it every day because it makes you sleepy. Or you may discover that eating fresh strawberries and raspberries at lunch is fine, but in the morning too many of them can spike your blood sugar and leave you with a headache.

SPECIFIC STRATEGIES FOR "MANAGING" YOUR LIFE AND YOUR DIET.

Remember what I said earlier: the elimination diet is temporary.

You want to get back to living a life of joy and stability, and part of that is eating what you like to eat! The idea is to find your "new normal". There are times when feeling a little unsettled may be worth it for an extraordinary meal or when you have a craving, but by having the knowledge of what you're getting into beforehand, you can make smarter, healthier choices that hand the power of how you feel *back* to you.

7

BEST PRACTICES FOR SUCCEEDING WITH AN ELIMINATION DIET

There are a lot of things to consider when beginning an elimination diet, but don't worry! There are plenty of us who have walked this path before you. Here's a collection of the best tips and strategies I've gathered from helping people through the elimination diet over the years.

#1 GET AT LEAST A WEEK'S WORTH OF GROCERIES & MEAL PLANS IN PLACE BEFORE BEGINNING.

As I mentioned in Phase 1, the last thing you want to do is walk into your kitchen hungry and not know what you can eat. Take the time to set yourself up — it's worth it. A lot of people even eat similar foods for the whole three week "cleaning" phase. The less barriers to eating healthy, the better. Whatever you need to do to make this easier on yourself, do it.

#2 CHOOSE A TIME WHEN YOU'RE MOST LIKELY TO STICK TO IT.

Don't plan it during a month of weddings, during the Christmas holidays, or when you have a big vacation coming up. Half the battle is not putting yourself in situations where social pressure will make you crack. If you're taking a romantic getaway to Savannah to eat all sorts of delicious shrimp and grits and seafood, maybe it's not the best time. Do you have a quiet month ahead of you? Jump in.

#3 DON'T MAKE ANY OTHER BIG CHANGES TO YOUR LIFE OR ROUTINE

Because the idea is to establish baselines and isolate what foods are causing different symptoms, you want to avoid changing your life and routine in any significant way. Here are some things you'll want to avoid while executing an elimination diet:

Significantly changing your exercise routine.

Starting a new exercise routine and the elimination diet at the same time isn't the best idea. Because this change in routine will affect your nutritional needs, it will make it more difficult to figure out what foods are making you feel what way and why.

New jobs or other possible stress triggers

If possible, try not to conduct the elimination diet during transitions of any sort. Stress can have powerful physical effects on the body, and we don't want to confuse those with what you're feeling from your elimination diet experiment. If you know you're leaving your job in the next month, consider holding off. Life will obviously get in the way of the most thorough and careful plans, but you should start this process with the mindset of not "rocking the boat".

Switching to vegetarianism or any other major nutritional switch.

The elimination diet is already a big enough nutritional change. Don't try to combine this with keto, paleo, or any other sort of change. Just focus on the elimination diet for now.

#4 DRINK AS MUCH WATER AS YOU CAN

When you stop eating foods that have been causing inflammation, it's natural for your body to get rid of water. To help manage this effect and make sure you don't get stuck with any unnecessary headaches, try drinking between 64oz & 128oz of water a day. I know it's a lot, but it really helps. I advise my clients to buy a reusable water bottle and keep it by their bed. Waking up and drinking a lot of water helps you wake up and reach your daily water goal faster.

#5 FOR THE EASIEST, SAFEST, AND MOST EFFICIENT WAY TO CONDUCT AN ELIMINATION DIET, WORK WITH A PROFESSIONAL.

You don't need a health professional to conduct an elimination diet, but they can really help. Going on an elimination diet is incredibly valuable and one of the smartest decisions you can make, but it's definitely easier when you don't have to do both the dieting and heavy-lifting in terms of thinking. Social accountability is also really powerful. The simple reminder that you have a scheduled talk with your nutritionist or functional wellness physician will help motivate you to stay on track. You can absolutely do this on your own, but my clients tell me all the time that it's so much easier with our check-ins & guidance.

It can also help to look at your past habits — is planning part of your personality? If you have a history of overplanning and love learning new systems, then you may be okay. If you know you need people to push you, then hiring a professional will make sure you finish what you started.

#6 SECOND GUESS YOUR EXISTING OPINIONS AND IDEAS OF WHAT FOODS ARE BAD FOR YOU.

It's very common for people to have ideas of what foods are bad for them & avoid them only to find that in fact it was a different food category that was causing the harm. Try to walk into this process with a clean mental slate. Some other things to note on food tracking...

Just because a food irritates you doesn't mean it's inherently *bad* and should be discarded for good, you may just have to adjust how much and when you eat it.

Do not alter or stop following any advice given to you by a medical professional. If you're allergic or have a medical condition that *requires* you to eat or not eat certain foods, do not change these! Simply modify the elimination diet as needed.

Don't get excited and call the tests early. Conversely, don't get down and call the diet early. You need five full days for each reintroduction to get reliable results. You can do it!

#7 BECOME A LABEL-READING NINJA.

At the beginning of the clean eating phase, you'll have to keep a close eye on labels for potential irritants. Many of the foods you think are fine may have preservatives or sugars in them — this goes for foods labeled as "healthy" and "organic" as well. Get in the habit of looking at the labels for any food you buy from the store. In general, the longer the ingredient list, the worse it is for you, and most frozen foods, canned soups, and preserved products will have suspect ingredients.

Here's what to watch out for on labels:

- **Added sugar and high fructose corn syrup.**
  If any product includes "added sugar", then it's a no-go. Natural sugars in some foods is just fine, but additions are something we want to avoid during the clean-eating phase.
- **Wheat**
- **Soy**
- **MSG**
- **Chicory root, inulin, fructo-oligosaccharides.**
- **Sorbitol, xylitol, or hydrogenated starch hydrolysates.**
- **Sodium nitrates/nitrites.**

- **Hydrogenated oils, aka trans fat.**
- **Artificial flavors and colors.**
- **Artificial sweeteners.**
- **Oils: Corn, vegetable, and soybean.**
- **Enriched wheat.**
- **Carrageenan.**

A rule to make things easier: If you can't pronounce the ingredient, it's probably bad! Stick to simple ingredient lists with words you recognize as much as possible.

NEXT STEPS AND FINAL WORDS

.

You now have everything you need to conduct a successful elimination diet, but there are a few more things I'd like to say. The first being, *you can do this*. The elimination diet is not easy, but nothing ever worth it is. You have the opportunity to potentially rid yourself of chronic bloating, gas, intestinal issues, headaches, fatigue... Isn't that worth the temporary inconvenience?

And you're already dealing with inconvenience in your daily life, right? The quality of life you want *is* achievable, even if it feels like some impossible hill you're climbing. Don't accept defeat — take the steps and try this elimination diet out. I promise it's worth your time.

Second, consider working with a doctor. If you want to make sure that you finish this and that you did it right, you can't replace professional guidance. And full disclosure, I'm a functional medicine doctor and elimination diet specialist who runs a health clinic called the Strong Health Institute. While we would love to help you through the elimination diet, we also recognize that it doesn't have to be us. You could work with anyone, but we have a proven system that has helped person after person finally achieve a quality of life they love. If you want to have all the heavy lifting handled for you, get the best app, materials, and resources given to you, and hop on weekly calls to make sure you're on track and doing everything as you should, then I'd love to help. We work locally in middle TN but also have clients all around the country who work with us virtually.

To get in touch, just email us at drstrong@stronghealthinstitute.com or get in touch on our website:

https://stronghealthinstitute.com/

Either way, I want this to be a win for you. You have everything you need to succeed. The next step is up to you.

Best of luck,

Todd M. Strong D.C. DACNB, CFMP, PAK

ABOUT THE AUTHOR

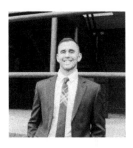

Todd M. Strong D.C. DACNB, CFMP, PAK is a graduate from Life University, the largest chiropractic college in the world, who has studied Applied Kinesiology, Functional Neurology, and Functional Medicine. While at Life University, he enrolled in outside courses of Applied Kinesiology earning over 400 hours of training and earning his Practitioner of Applied Kinesiology certification.

Dr. Strong has completed extensive training in functional medicine training. He earned his Certified Functional Medicine Practitioner training through FMU. This included over 300 hours of nutrition, lab interpretation, program design, and advanced biochemistry. He is also a member of the Kalish Institute, this program constantly refines functional medicine protocols, lab interpretation, and research to provide the best practices and education. He is also a graduate of a course at the Carrick Institute, which dealt with brain-based rehabilitation for a multitude of neurological conditions. This course required 300 hours of clinical neuroscience academia, rehab modalities, and case interpretations. Along with his functional neurology training, he has also completed 150 hours of vestibular rehabilitation training.

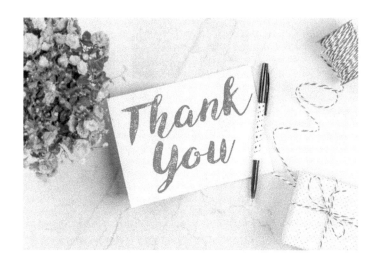

It would mean a lot if you took a minute of your time to leave a review. It really helps small clinic owners like me and can just be a few short sentences.

CLICK HERE

OTHER BOOKS YOU'LL ENJOY

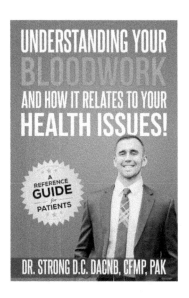

Link Here: https://www.amazon.com/dp/B08CPB4TQJ/

A FREE GIFT TO OUR READERS!

And don't forget to get your complimentary Elimination Diet starter pack!

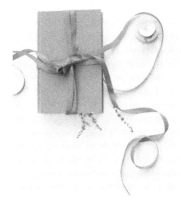

Download the checklists, food diary templates, and more that will make your Elimination Diet journey so much easier!

Visit this link:

https://stronghealthinstitute.activehosted.com/f/19

ADDITIONAL RESOURCES AND
RESEARCH:

Many of the statements and claims made in this book are backed by peer-reviewed research. If you would dig deeper into the science behind the elimination diet, here are a few resources and studies to refer to:

https://pubmed.ncbi.nlm.nih.gov/12532668/

https://www.sciencedirect.com/science/article/abs/pii/S0091674912026449

https://www.ncbi.nlm.nih.gov/pmc/articles/PMC3970830

https://www.tandfonline.com/doi/abs/10.1080/07315724.2006.10719567

https://link.springer.com/article/10.1186/s13601-016-0115-x

https://www.functionalmedicineuniversity.com/public/976.cfm

https://www.functionalmedicineuniversity.com/public/806.cfm

https://www.nature.com/articles/1600990

https://www.healthline.com/nutrition/elimination-diet#section1

https://stronghealthinstitute.com/we-are-having-new-department-added-to-us-3/

Lightning Source UK Ltd.
Milton Keynes UK
UKHW020707080321
379980UK00016B/2460